Fung Shwe

Tips from the Fun

MW01292905

Table of Contents

Introduction By Dr. Fung 2

Foreword Megan and Angel Ramos 3

  About The Authors 6

    Acknowledgements 6

      Disclaimer 7

Fasting Regimens by Sandy T Rodriguez 8

  Fat Fasting by Sandy T Rodriguez 12

John's Story by John Clary 16

Quick Dietary Guide by Juan Peralta 21

The Importance Of Hydration By Pete Kaye 23

  The Fat Within By Pete Kaye 25

    Sleep, Hormones and the "Faster's High" By Pete Kaye 26

    Autophagy by Pete Kaye 29

      All about Protein by Pete Kaye 30

Ketogenic Diets by Gina More Minis 31

  What About Cholesterol 37

    To Snack or Not To Snack by Gina More Minis 41

    The Perils Of Sweeteners by Gina More Minis 43

      Weight Stalling By Gina More Minis 45

Testimonials by Fung Shweigh Group Members 51

Recipes 54

  Gina's 1 Week Sample Menu By Gina More Minis 71

Resources 76

Introduction

By Dr. Jason Fung

Fasting is one of the oldest dietary interventions known to mankind. Our bodies have evolved mechanisms to adapt to periods without food. When food became plentiful, religions played a large role in keeping this fasting tradition. This was not because they thought it was harmful, but instead, believed it to have an important role in keeping the body healthy. This explains how it is often referred to as a 'cleanse' or 'detoxification'.

Fasting is an important technique that enables you to regain control over your own health. However, it is not always easy and certainly not always fun. This is why online support groups like Fung Shweigh are so important. You can draw on the collective wisdom and experience of others just like yourself who are willing to make the effort to get healthier.

-Dr. Jason Fung

Foreword

By Megan Ramos, Program Director at Intensive Dietary Management Clinic (IDM) and Angel Ramos, Director of the Male Metabolic Program at Intensive Dietary Management Clinic (IDM.

Dr. Jason Fung and I cannot thank the administrators and moderators of the Facebook Group, Fung Shweigh, enough for their dedication and support. The Fung Shweigh Facebook Group provides a safe place for many of our Intensive Dietary Management (IDM) participants and followers to go and seek support, encouragement and sound advice from likeminded individuals. We are so grateful that this group is available to help spread our message.

One of the most overwhelming aspects of adapting to this new lifestyle is the fact that there is so much contradictory information out there. The administrators and moderators of Fung Shweigh do their best to make sure that the information provided on the group page is streamlined and not contradictory. The group does a tremendous job at making sure the information is clear based on the philosophies and principles established by Dr. Jason Fung and myself when we co-founded the IDM program in 2013.

One of the things I enjoy the most about the Fung Shweigh group is the fact that they allow members to engage in sensible debate rather than personal attacks based on disagreeing beliefs. Each person has unique metabolic issues. Some people can only have water and salt when they fast. Some people have poor mineral and electrolyte adsorption and need to take a few extra training wheels during their fasting periods. What works well for one person may not work at all for another person. What is safe for one person may not be safe at all for another. The administrators and moderations of the group understand there is no "one-size-fits-all" model. They ensure that each member is free to state what they are doing during their fasting periods without being ridiculed by another individual since they are doing something slightly or dramatically different from them.

I started my own personal fasting journey nearly 6 years ago after struggling to lose weight and manage diabetes, fatty liver disease, polycystic ovarian syndrome, cancerous cells and a birth defect in my heart. I had no support when I first started fasting. My friends thought I was psychotic. My father is a lawyer and I was

3

convinced he and my mother were going to try to get some sort of power of attorney over me because they thought I was mad. Of course, I worked with Jason day-in and day-out, but we were both so busy at work. I really struggled without the support. I wish there was a group like Fung Shweigh where I could have gone and sought out the assistance of peers going through the same struggles as I was.

I enjoy how the group always tries to rally people together to do group fasts and various feasting challenges as well. Seeing this motivates me, and I often join in for the challenges. The best way to succeed at this lifestyle is to constantly mix things up, and I love how the Fung Shweigh team is always encouraging their members to challenge themselves in various ways. Like myself, most of us do not have support from our family members, colleagues and peers within our own personal communities. Fung Shweigh allows for communities of likeminded people to gather and participate in succeeding in this lifestyle together.

-Megan J. Ramos

Angel Ramos

I first met my wife and Intensive Dietary Management (IDM) co-founded and director, Megan Ramos, well into her fasting journey. She had reversed her diabetes, fatty liver, polycystic ovarian syndrome, and she had also lost over 60 pounds at this point. I only knew my wife as a very healthy and spunky individual.

The year before meeting Megan I was traveling in Europe with some friends. Our vacation was well documented with thousands of ridiculous photos from across the continent. Upon our return home, my very best friends took me aside and told me I needed to lose weight. They were genuinely concerned for my health and wellbeing. I had no idea how much weight I had really gained until I saw myself in the pictures from our trip. That was not the person I saw looking back at me in the mirror. I started carb-loading and working out. I lost some weight, but I was always hungry. I wasn't gaining the kind of strength I had sought out either. No matter how many protein shakes I consumed, my muscles just didn't grow. I was going at it non-stop for months and only lost about 25 lbs.

Megan and I started dating in the fall of 2014. She was living in Toronto, Canada, and I was living in the San Francisco Bay area of California. I knew Megan was heavily focused on disease prevention in her career, but as our relationship progressed she opened up to me about her struggles with metabolic syndrome and told me about her journey with intermittent fasting. As a scientist myself, I was extremely curious and went to the IDM website to learn more. It all made sense. It all made perfect sense. Part of me felt like such an idiot for not knowing better, because I should have known better.

I started fasting intermittently for 24-hours and even trying so prolonged periods of fasting. I was more than willing to embrace the bacon and egg lifestyle too. I figured you had to marry any woman who insisted on eating bacon and eggs all the time, and within a year we were married. I was down a total of 70 lbs. by our wedding day. I lost 50 lbs. in half the time it took me to lose 25 lbs. just by fasting, not snacking, and eating a lot of bacon.

I am honored to be able to have the opportunity to manage the Intensive Dietary Management's Male Metabolic Program to help other men achieve the same results that I have. Weight-loss for men is very different than that of women. The effects of fasting can be very different for men as well. It is a real privilege to work with these gentlemen and help them regain control of their weight and health again.

-Angel Ramos

About The Authors

Gina More Minis is a home maker that improved her health and lost one hundred and eighty pounds using a low carb, high fat, ketogenic diet with intermittent fasting.

Sandy Tucker Rodriguez is in the Intensive Dietary Management Program, has improved her health and lost weight with diet and fasting. She is the founder and owner of the Fung Shweigh for Diabetes/Metabolic Issues Facebook Group, inspired by Dr. Fung. Its focus is on teaching, helping and supporting those on their journey to metabolic health.

Authors' Note: We decided to write this book from the perspective of personal experiences during this journey. We are not doctors, but our stories will be valuable to others who are fat and sick.

Acknowledgements

A very special thank you is given to our contributors, Pete Kaye and John Clary, who are moderators of the Fung Shweigh Facebook group. Thank you to Juan Peralta, Gina's husband, who has also improved his health with the help of this group and his extensive research.

A heart-felt thank you is given to our group members, who have given their testimonials.

This book is dedicate to all of our members. We wouldn't be here without you!

Disclaimer

The information contained in this book is not intended or implied to be a substitute for professional medical advice, diagnosis or treatment. All content, including text, graphics, images and information, contained on or available through this book is for general information purposes only. **NEVER DISREGARD PROFESSIONAL MEDICAL ADVICE OR DELAY SEEKING MEDICAL TREATMENT BECAUSE OF SOMETHING YOU HAVE READ OR ACCESSED THROUGH THIS BOOK.**

Do not attempt a fasting regimen or a fat fast if you are on any type of medication or have any pre-existing medical condition, without first seeking medical supervision. Fasting, including fat fasting, can drop blood glucose and blood pressure so rapidly, that it can be dangerous. Discuss the information in this book with your healthcare provider first, before implementation.

The Fung Shweigh Fasting Tips and its materials are not intended to treat, diagnose, cure or prevent any disease or ailment. All content on this book is intended for educational purposes only. Always seek the advice of your personal physician or healthcare provider before beginning any new diet, exercise regime or wellness routine.

The information contained in this book is to be used as a discussion guide with your doctor.

Fasting Regimens

By Sandy Tucker Rodriguez

Sandy's before and after:

Before: In 2002, my weight was 227 lbs. I tried losing weight on low carb, but the weight came back. I had high blood pressure and my fasting blood glucose was 112.

After: As of today, I have lost 32 inches. I now weigh 195 pounds. My A1C decreased to 5.4 from 6.2, and my fasting glucose is now 88. My fasting insulin went from 14.5 to 10.5.

My journey is very similar to others. One day I went to the doctor for my yearly exam. My doctor ordered routine blood work for me. When the lab work came back, my doctor looked over them and said my cholesterol was great but my blood glucose was starting to rise. It was 112. She said I had the beginning symptom of insulin resistance. The only thing to do was to keep an eye on it. She would perform a re-test in 6 months. I was disturbed by the results. My blood glucose had never been over 99 at any time and that high number of 112 scared me to death. I was even more disturbed by the "keep an eye on it" recommendation. Just what was that supposed to do?

I went home but decided that instead of keeping an eye on it, I was going to do some research. I searched insulin resistance, high blood sugar and diabetes. What I read wasn't very positive and it scared me even more than I already was. I told myself I had to do something about this now. There was no way I wanted to be put on lifelong medications. Now that I knew what it was, it was time for me to research how to stop it.

I always enjoyed reading blogs and Facebook pages so I went there. One page after another, searching to see what I could find to help me lower this high blood glucose before my next doctor appointment. I eventually came across this doctor named Dr. Jason Fung on his website. I watched his webinars. I learned all I could about this doctor in the next 4 months. His protocol appeared so easy. It was fasting.

It sounds pretty simple right? Eat when you are hungry, stop when you are full. If you are not hungry, you do not have to eat. Learn to listen to your body. This is where intermittent fasting plays its role. The less we eat, the more fasting we will do, and that will help lower our insulin.

What I learned about Dr. Fung, that stood out was that: All I had to do was eat less and fast more.

I was already on a low carb diet, so all I had to do was learn to fast. I first read Dr. Fung's articles and watched his webinars online. I started with "The Aetiology of Obesity", a six part series, which is available for free on YouTube and explains obesity in its entirety. I would recommend anyone to start with "How to Cure Diabetes". My two favorite topics are the video, "Part 3 – Trial by Diet" from "The Aetiology of Obesity" and the article, "The Fasting Advantage - Part 14".

The best way to tackle a problem is to learn everything you can from it. You need to understand its root causes. Dr. Fung's simple and detailed explanation opened my eyes to this fact. I had to restore my body's homeostasis by allowing it to fast. It cannot be easier. Fasting simply means to not eat and only drink water.

Sandy's Way of Fasting

There are many fasting regimens Dr. Fung recommends. Simply choose the right one for your lifestyle. This allows you to sustain and consistently practice it. Dr. Fung recommends a fasting regimen no less than 12 hours per day. From there, you can choose the regimen that will help you achieve your goals. You can choose a daily, intermittent or extended fasting regimen.

- Daily fasting: A fasting window between 12 to 20 hours per day
- Intermittent fasting: Eat every other day
- Extended fasting: Fast for multiple days at a time (E.g., Many people like to eat during the week and fast all weekend. Others prefer to eat on the weekends and fast during the week.)

During your fasting window, you should only have water, salt, coffee, tea, bone broth and/or mineral water. Cream is allowed in the coffee or tea. Eventually, water consumption alone will be tolerable as your "fasting muscle" becomes stronger.

Armed with this information, I was ready to begin! I started fasting. I chose an extended three day fast and jumped right in. The experience was liberating. I had plenty of time to easily focus on other things besides eating and did not feel any adverse effects.

I began to routinely fast and implement different regimens. When I follow a 16-18 hour fast, my eating window is 6-8 hours. I can accommodate 2 meals during this time. I also follow a 36 hour fast, which consists of fasting for an entire day and eating 3 meals the next day.

I joined the IDM Program. Being on the IDM Program, under supervision by Megan, I am allowed to undergo extended fasts. I make sure to obtain the required blood work and that my doctor is aware of my fasting.

Fact: You can apply a fasting regimen to any diet. Even if you are vegetarian, fruitarian, vegan, etc., you can benefit from fasting. The most important thing is to find a regimen that works best for your diet and lifestyle.

Sandy's Way of Eating:

I decided to learn more about the eating aspect because I felt adequately familiar with fasting. My goal was to lose weight. I had to find the proper balance of eating and fasting. Diet and fasting influence each other, and choosing the right diet is as important as choosing a fasting regimen. So, my next step was to find out what to eat and when to eat. Below is what I discovered.

I love vegetables, so I found a way to make this diet work for me. I learned from my research that I needed to add fat to my vegetables. It had to be healthy, like coconut oil, butter and bacon fat. I love fish. I added salmon and tuna to my meals.

I began eating lunch at around 12am and dinner at 4pm. I found it's best to prepare my food for the week to prevent poor food choices.

The weight began to drop. In three months, my weight dropped to 210 lbs. from 227 lbs. Then, I plateaued. So I opened a Facebook group for encouragement. I also contacted Dr. Fung and asked him if I could add his name to the group. He approved. So, Fung Shweigh was born. Since creating the group, I learned that fasting provided benefits beyond weight loss. Examples include more energy, focus and less inflammation.

To this day, I am still working to improve my health. I weigh daily and measure my waist circumference every 3 months. I monitor my blood glucose about 3 times per day and track my blood pressure as well. This keeps me accountable and aware of any changes I need to make.

Fact: The body doesn't count calories. Dr. Fung states, "The body's currency is not calories, its insulin". The cycle is of feast and famine, not of dieting and not dieting. The body needs to feel completely satisfied when it eats and deplete its stores when it fasts, before it eats again. It's what signals the hormones to be released in pulses, and keeps you lean independent of caloric consumption.

When you fast, eat nothing. This signals your body to drop insulin and release fat stores. Metabolism speeds up to find food. If you're still eating, but limiting your calories, then you're on caloric restriction or C.R.A.P. (Caloric Restriction as Primary). This tells your body to slow down its metabolism because there is not enough food.

Why Sandy Fasts:

1. For resilience against many chronic diseases
2. To curb starch and sugar cravings
3. To stabilize blood glucose and insulin levels
4. To repair damaged cells
5. To reduce A1C

Fat Fasting

By Sandy Tucker Rodriguez

A fat fast is a jacked up ketogenic diet. It consists of eating primarily fatty foods. It is used to break the starch and sugar habit, as well as to help lower blood glucose. It can also help you break a weight-loss plateau and become fat adapted, whereby fat is used as fuel. I came up with a Fat Fast idea called the Bacon, Olive and Avocado fast (B.O.A.). The goal is to have these three foods for 3-5 days prior to a zero calorie fast. A fat fast prior to a zero calorie fast helps me fast longer with less cravings and hunger. The additional Himalayan salt is beneficial and important for hydration.

Fat fasting has been used for many years. I came across fat fasting in books about fasting, but I never tried it until I enrolled in the IDM Program. Megan suggested it to me for the reduction of ghrelin, a hunger signaling hormone.

Fact: Glycogen stores in the liver decrease 12 to 16 hours into a fast. This suggests the duration is sufficient to trigger autophagy. Autophagy or "self-eating" is the main mechanism to eliminate intracellular pathogens. During this process, damaged proteins, bacteria, viruses and other germs are broken down and "digested". Their constituent parts are reused by the cell to make new, useful proteins and organelles. Autophagy is suppressed during eating and digestion.

Sandy's B.O.A.

- Bacon - As much as you want (5 to 12 slices a day)
- Olives - As much as you want (15-30)
- Avocados - 2 per day
- Eat to satiety (2 meals per day)

I find that on day 1 I can eat a pound of bacon, but by day 4, I reduce the amount of bacon I eat. A week on the B.O.A. fast leads me to a zero calorie fast, consisting of water (mineral), salt and tea.

Why Avocados, Bacon and Olives?

- Avocados are nutrient-dense and a great source of fat. They also contain many minerals. These include potassium and magnesium. Along with sodium, the combination helps keep our electrolytes in balance.
- Olives are a great source of fat or nature's "fat bombs", containing anti-oxidants, oleic acid and polyphenols. Black olives contain Vitamin E.
- Bacon is high in fat and omega 3 fatty acids. It contains protein as well, while remaining carbohydrate free. This makes it the perfect choice for the BOA.

Sandy's 0 Calorie Fast Example:

- Unlimited water with sea salt, lemon slices and/or apple cider vinegar
- Unlimited mineral water
- Unlimited, unsweetened tea, hot or cold
- Bone or vegetable broth, up to 3 cups per day (Dr. Fung's book - The Obesity Code has a bone broth recipe.)

My quick vegetable broth recipe – any above ground vegetables, greens, herbs and spices, cooked in a slow cooker for 8-12 hours

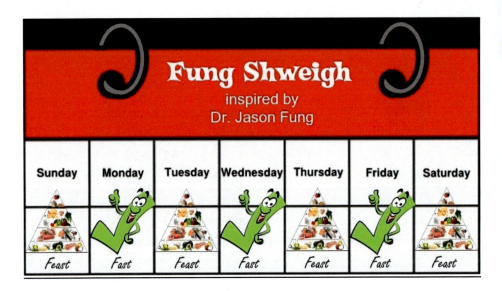

Graph is courtesy of Manny Gomez

Sandy's Favorite Meals Menu:

Day 1 –

•	Breakfast: Bacon (4-6 slices), 1 avocado with salt, tea and water.

•	Lunch: green salad with cucumbers, radishes, cherry tomatoes, olives, sunflower seeds, feta cheese with apple cider vinegar and extra virgin olive oil. This salad can be topped with salmon, tuna or bacon. You can also add pecans and an avocado. Mineral water.

•	Dinner: Salmon cooked with green peppers and onions, coleslaw, cabbage dish with butter or green beans and bacon. Water and tea.

Day 2 –

•	Breakfast: Bacon (4-6 slices), avocado with salsa, tea and water.

•	Lunch: Grilled chicken with a green salad, radishes, cucumbers, broccoli, olives and feta cheese. Tea and water.

•	Dinner: Big green salad, romaine, spinach leaves, mushrooms, raw cauliflower, walnuts, cherry tomatoes, green peppers, green onion and tuna or salmon.

Day 3 –

- Breakfast: 1 avocado stuffed with green salad, feta cheese, pecans, olives and homemade mayonnaise. Tea and water.

- Lunch: 1 avocado, raw cauliflower with a ranch-style dressing. Mineral water.

- Dinner: Cooked, mashed cauliflower with bacon, butter-grilled chicken with green peppers, green onions and mozzarella cheese.

*Himalayan salt was used liberally.

Sandy's 11 Fasting Tips

1. Prepare mentally by reading the IDM articles before fasting.
2. Plan your fast and keep a journal.
3. Keep busy - go walking, do gardening or read a book.
4. Drink plenty of water throughout the day.
5. Re-feeding - Start with 1/2 an avocado or vegetable soup 30 minutes before a meal.
6. Get organized - Buy mineral water, tea, ingredients for a vegetable broth or soup before fasting.
7. The best fasting regimen is the one that works for you and your lifestyle.
8. If your current fasting schedule no longer works for you, change it.
9. When should I worry about electrolytes? Always
10. Feeling cold while fasting suggests you should consume more fat on eating days
11. You may be losing inches even when you are not losing pounds, so make sure to measure your waist, hips and abs.

John's Story

By John Clary

I was a chubby kid, not too fat, but big enough that my mom had to buy me "husky" sized clothes. I grew up on a farm and there wasn't much processed food around the house but we definitely ate a lot of starchy foods – macaroni, potatoes, bread. Many people on my mother's side of the family, including my mother, were overweight or obese.

Eating habits at home weren't the best. There was always an after-school snack and a bedtime snack in addition to three full meals a day. Fried potatoes almost every night. Homemade donuts and cakes. Ice cream before bed. That was our normal.

I stayed chubby until I was about 12 years old and then the weight started to come on quickly. By that time we had moved to the suburbs and with that came easy access to convenience stores and fast food. I would beg, borrow and steal to get the food I wanted. Sweets, sure, I liked the cookies and cakes but I was crazy for savory food like burgers and fries, pizza, mac and cheese.

This was a terrible time in my life, many traumatic things were going on and my food was one of the few things I had control over. No doubt I was eating for emotional reasons. By the time I reached high school I was wearing size 44 pants. And I kept growing. Clothes became difficult to find, only through mail order. I was teased and bullied throughout high school, even by my own "friends". It's a wonder I stayed on through graduation.

I went off to college and was able to start a new life there which I enjoyed immensely. I made a lot of friends in my dorm and through activities. I also enjoyed the cafeteria food. Unlimited amounts of favorite foods and all I had to do was show up. At some time during college I required size 54 pants and 3 XL shirts.

I had a somewhat normal life for such an obese person, at least I thought I did. I finished college and started a working life. It was a lot different than college. I found out it was a lot harder out there. It seemed like I was always alone. No one wanted to be around a big fat guy. For the first time, I started to think that losing weight might be a good thing. Strangely, it hadn't really occurred to me before.

I was in my late 20's, no social life, just working, watching TV and eating. I was very unhappy. My mother mailed me some literature about Overeaters Anonymous (OA) and it sounded interesting. Somehow I mustered up the courage to attend a meeting and it was the beginning of a big change. I clicked well with the program and people wanted to help me. I followed a way of eating that reduced starchy foods and sugar and required me to weigh and measure my food. I started to lose weight and with that, become happier. I'm not sure what my starting weight was at the time but I estimate it at 400 pounds.

Following OA wasn't always easy, I went through binge periods every few weeks but kept coming back. After a couple of years I had lost about 150 pounds.

By this time, my social life really picked up and I found myself dating a woman who would later become my wife. She had struggled with overeating herself and we found ourselves enabling each other. Over the next few years I gained back all of my weight and she became morbidly obese also.

We had children and I felt that I needed to get my weight under control so that I could live and be a father to them. OA didn't seem to work for me anymore, it just seemed like a gimmick. Like many people, I was trying to eat low-fat and move more. I forgot about cutting out the starchy foods and sugar. Out of desperation, I went under the knife and had Roux-en-Y Gastric Bypass Surgery. I remember the shame I felt when I was weighed before surgery and the industrial type scale read 424.

After surgery it was constant pain. The weight started coming off but after about three months, 75 lbs. loss, it stopped. I noticed that I could eat more. I noticed that I could eat sweets. An endoscopy revealed that the staples in my stomach pouch had come loose and my stomach was just as large as if I hadn't had the surgery at all. It wasn't long before I was back up to about 400 pounds. My wife wasn't far behind me. We lived a life filled with junk food, fast food, restaurant food and two-liter bottles of soda. I was diagnosed with Type 2 Diabetes and was so ashamed, I never talked about it with anyone and I just took my pills and shots. I was also on statins, blood pressure medication and meds for acid reflux.

After 14 years of marriage, we divorced. This was about the time that The Biggest Loser premiered and I thought I found the answer. I would go through periods of calorie restriction and lots of exercise and lose 50-70 pounds, feel great but always went back to my old habits and regained the weight. This happened every year or two. I could not understand why I could not stick with it and was constantly beating myself up about it.

At the beginning of 2016 my employer started a wellness program and I decided to get on board. I weighed in at 396 pounds. I read about the Paleo way of eating with whole natural foods and tried to incorporate changes into the way I ate. I read about low carbohydrate diets and tried to use some of those methods. I started losing a little and was feeling better but was still white-knuckling it, being driven by food cravings. I would have the worst episodes in the evenings, pacing the kitchen, looking in the pantry and refrigerator, feeling like I just HAD to have something! Sometimes I could resist, sometimes I could not.

I spent time every day reading articles about food and dieting, perusing recipes, looking for answers. I found a blog that mentioned Dr. Jason Fung and his work with diabetics and was led to the Intensive Dietary Management website. I read everything I could and decided to order his book. I was told that everything in the book was on the website but I am so glad I bought the book because it was written in a way that things were explained logically.

April 20, 2016 was the day I read The Obesity Code and I read it in one day. First, I went to the back of the book and read the appendix to find out what I was supposed to do and then started at the beginning to understand why. It was exciting to learn that it was possible to reverse my diabetes. The medications I was on were losing effectiveness and my doctor said insulin injections were next.

The way Dr. Fung explained how insulin worked was a revelation to me. I remember reading that passage in the book and thinking IT'S NOT MY FAULT!! I had an answer to the WHY question I had my entire life. Why can't I control my food? Why can't I say no? Why the obsession and compulsion?

I now understood that I had a hormonal problem, one that I probably have had my entire life. Insulin, leptin, ghrelin – they were all working against me! My metabolism was deranged!

Insulin. Now I understood why I needed to limit my eating opportunities to meals with no snacks. Fasting? I was one of those people who ate at least three meals a day with plenty of snacks. Breakfast is the most important meal of the day! Miss a meal? No way!!

I decided that I would try what Dr. Fung suggested and skip breakfast, having only black coffee. That would give me about a 16 hour fast. This was probably the first time I had ever drank black coffee but I managed it. Lunch time came around and I felt good so I did what Dr. Fung suggested and pushed through. The same thing happened at dinner.

I woke up the next day and had my black coffee again. I felt pretty good so I kept fasting. During this second day I got a little foggy headed but didn't feel bad. By the next day my mind felt sharp and focused. Ketosis! I felt amazed that I could go three entire days without eating anything!

Eating lunch and dinner only, with no snacking, became my regular routine and I have followed that since April 2016. There have been times where I have fasted for an extended period, as long as seven days. I'm a bit of a purist when I fast, I consume only black coffee and water plus electrolytes. I have nothing against bone broth or a couple of teaspoons of cream if someone chooses to use them, I just feel think they are not necessary for me.

I was faithfully tracking everything I ate on My Fitness Pal and I continued eating what I thought was low carbohydrate, 100-150 grams of carbohydrate a day, until I discovered a website about the zero carbohydrate way of eating -- only foods from the animal kingdom. Then I learned about the ketogenic diet and how keeping my carbohydrates under 20 grams a day would keep me in fat-burning ketosis. Once I started following this, my food cravings went away entirely. Food became my fuel and although I could still enjoy what I ate, I did not obsess over it. It's been well over a year since I had any kind of binge or went off my plan. I now know I have a carbohydrate intolerance.

Within about six weeks of beginning intermittent fasting and reducing carbohydrates my blood glucose readings normalized. Instead of morning readings as high as 180, they were around 120. Shortly afterwards I discontinued taking Bydureon injections, statins, and meds for blood pressure and acid reflux.

As of this writing in June 2017, my A1C is 5.4 – right in the middle of the normal range. After I eat a meal my glucose goes up a few points and an hour or two later it is back to normal. I consider myself cured of Type 2 Diabetes. As a welcome side effect, I have lost 135 pounds. I think I have an additional 40 pounds to go. I'm not quite sure because I have never been a normal weight. I'll know when I get there.

After a lifetime of struggling, I found the solution for me was to simply change what and when I eat.

-John Clary

Quick Dietary Guide

By Juan Peralta

<hr>

Juan's before and after:

Before: In 2012, my weight was 346 lbs. I was having symptoms of neuropathy and vascular disease in my lower extremities. I had an enlarged heart, high blood pressure and atherosclerotic plaque in my carotid arteries. I was also having debilitating neurological symptoms.

After: Today, I have reversed my high blood pressure and dropped my weight to 209 lbs. My neuropathy, vascular disease and atherosclerosis have improved significantly, up to 60%. My neurological symptoms have tapered down.

<hr>

- Choose organic, non-GMO foods when possible. Avoid foods containing antibiotics and/or hormones.
- Improve your digestion with raw, unfiltered, apple cider vinegar with the 'mother'.
- Eat foods that provide important nutrients and anti-oxidants, such as pasture-raised eggs, grass-fed dairy, avocados, raw almonds and broccoli.
- Eat high quality proteins, such as grass-fed and finished beef, wild-caught seafood, pole-caught skipjack or yellow fin tuna and free-range poultry, such as turkey. Don't overcook.
- Only choose coconut oil, avocado oil, extra virgin olive oil, clarified butter or ghee, grass-fed imported butter and/or tallow to prepare foods. Don't overheat.
- Avoid all grains, such as corn, wheat, rice and associated inflammatory seed oils, which may be found in processed foods and supplements.
- Avoid ingredients you can't decipher, pronounce or buy readily at a farmer's market. Avoid foods with added fructose, sugar and/or chemical substitutes listed in the ingredients section.
- Implement intermittent fasting of up to 12 hours per day.

Juan's Top 10 Healthy Fats

- Coconut Oil
- Ghee
- Butter
- Macadamia Oil
- Cocoa Butter
- Lard
- Tallow
- Palm Oil (Red)
- Extra Virgin Olive Oil
- Avocado Oil

Fact: Combining fat with sugar is the worst thing anyone can do. When you mix fat and sugar, the body tries to burn sugar first and fails due to the overload, so the sugar is converted into fat. Furthermore, all of the fat you eat is stored while your body continues to process the sugar. The key to improving insulin resistance is to deplete excess sugar stores and avoid further consumption.

The Importance of Hydration

By Pete Kaye

Pete's before and after:

Before: In 2003, I had a stent inserted in my left anterior descending cardiac artery (a.k.a. the widow maker). In 2006, I was diagnosed with malignant renal cell carcinoma, stage 3, and the remedy was to remove the affected kidney. I pursued a low fat diet to hopefully stabilize and improve my health with no benefit. Instead, I had two additional stents inserted in the same artery. By 2014, I was diagnosed as pre-diabetic at 320 lbs. That's when I began adopting a different plan of action and a low carbohydrate/high fat diet instead.

After: Fast forward to today and all of my blood tests have improved significantly. My lipid panel, inflammatory markers and blood pressure improved. I reduced my medications to two, instead of three, and at lower doses. Best of all, my remaining kidney function improved, which is not common.

So, how do you hydrate? Well, you drink plenty of water, right? Of course.

Hydration is vital because fasting drops your insulin levels significantly. Insulin retains water and therefore water is lost during fasting. With water loss comes the depletion of important electrolytes, replenished with hydration. However, a side-effect of excessive hydration is excessive urination. The minerals depleted as a result are sodium, potassium and magnesium.

During a fast, many people lose a lot of weight. Others lose less weight. Let's take a look.

Those Who Lose A Lot Of Weight (Quickly):

If you fast and begin to dehydrate, you will likely lose about 10 lbs. of weight in 10 days. But is this a good thing? If you are dehydrated and eat again, you will almost certainly regain half of it back. This is another reason to keep your electrolytes in check.

Many other things can happen as a result of dehydration. Lightheadedness, tachycardia and general malaise are some examples of common symptoms. So, was a net weight loss of about 5 lbs. worth the effort? Unlikely.

Those Who Lose Less Weight (Slowly):

As you fast, you should add beneficial salt to your coffee or (sparkling, mineral) water. You should also consume natural sources of potassium, as instructed by your doctor. Another way to do this is to use Lite Salt, a U.S. brand product, containing equal portions of sodium chloride and potassium chloride. Alternately, you can use Cream of Tartar, which is potassium bicarbonate.

The third electrolyte is magnesium. I supplement with a 400 IU tablet daily. This will yield a slower, steady weight loss of about 5 lbs. in 10 days.

The net effect is the same in both cases.

Many people want to lose a lot of weight for obvious reasons. To do this, they intentionally avoid salt. This is because salt triggers water retention and slower weight loss. This is risky because it makes dehydration harmfully worse for you.

I follow the slow weight loss method, consuming up to 3 liters of water per day.

I also drink coffee liberally during my water fasts. Because coffee is a diuretic, just like the extended fasts, I do the following. For every cup of caffeinated coffee I drink, I drink two cups of water. This way, weight gain will be minimal and the risk of an emergency room visit is significantly reduced.

The Fat Within

By Pete Kaye

We have three kinds of fats in our bodies.

Subcutaneous fat: These fatty deposits sit right under the skin and they are generally harmless.

Visceral fat: This is fat that surrounds the major organs, like the liver, stomach, intestines and kidneys. It is the one we see in obese patients with metabolic syndrome.

But there is one more kind of fat we have. It is called **ectopic fat.** Ectopic fat is defined by excess adipose tissue in locations not classically associated with adipose tissue storage. This is the fat Dr. Fung speaks of when he tells us about fatty liver, fatty pancreas, fatty musculature and fatty heart.

Luckily for us, lowering insulin and fasting eliminates all three of these types of fat!

Sleep, Hormones and the "Faster's High"

By Pete Kaye

Some common issues that are seen frequently, especially during a fast, is trouble sleeping and higher blood glucose readings in the morning. While most of us know this is not a biggie, why does it happen?

As we sleep, at about 4AM, a set of hormones are released in anticipation of our waking. What are they and why do they have this power to upset us?

Human Growth Hormone (HGH) is typically secreted during sleep and is one of the "counter-regulatory" hormones to insulin. HGH along with cortisol and adrenaline tell the body to increase the availability of glucose – so it counters the effect of insulin. High doses of HGH or cortisol will produce higher blood sugars. These hormones are typically secreted in pulses just before waking during the 'counter-regulatory surge'. These hormones can affect sleep.

When I am water fasting, I have sleep issues. I am awakened in the middle of the night. Most of the time, it occurs after 4-5 hours of sleep. It is usually good restful sleep, and so when it happens, it is time to turn on the coffee maker. There is no use trying to get back to sleep for me. But rather this time has become a productive "quiet time" for me. I'll usually use this time to do work on the computer or catch up on my reading. Even my pet Greyhounds love this one-on-one time, as I need to stroke their warm furry bodies to help quiet down these counter regulatory hormones. This is also the time of the day when my blood pressure is highest. I think it's because of the human growth hormone and norepinephrine which are released during an extended fast.

There are other hormones at work here too. At about the 36 hour point of a water/coffee fast, I get surges of hormones that give me a slight euphoric feeling. These are also counter regulatory hormones. In this instance, it is a class of hormones called the catecholamines. These are adrenaline, noradrenaline, epinephrine and norepinephrine. For me, they hit at the 36 hour point. I have learned to deal productively with them as well. Along with the hormones comes a euphoric, high energy feeling for me. I have heard some others who dislike this feeling. But for me, I have learned to love it and look forward to it. This is the best time to exercise. In fact, I personally call this my "Faster's High". For those who are frightened by this, try to work with it. I have, and I love it!

Remember that all hormones exhibit "pulsatile" secretion to prevent the development of resistance. Insulin, leptin, HGH, adrenaline; all these hormones are released the same way, albeit maybe at different frequencies. Where we get in trouble is when these "pulsatile" secretions become constant, and then we call them "hyper" secretions. This is bad. When we cause any hormone to be pulsed too frequently (a good example is insulin) then we become resistant to their effect.

Fast on, my friends!

Why Pete Fasts:

1. Weight loss – Primary reason for fasting.
2. Disease mitigation – We know fasting triggers autophagy. Along with its sister process of apoptosis, cancer and diseases of aging are kept in check. As a former cancer patient, I do not want to relapse. As a coronary artery disease patient, I want to improve endothelial function and blood flow.
3. Appetite control – Already under control with a ketogenic diet.
4. Strength and attainment of lean body mass – I added a mild aerobics class three days a week and mild weight lifting to my exercise routine. I incorporated muscle resistance training. As my muscle mass increased, my fat mass decreased from 48% to 31%. This is important at age 65.
5. Less (and hopefully no more) reliance on medications – When I started to follow Dr. Fung's advice and lose weight, I monitored my daily blood pressure. When I started, I was on four high-dose blood pressure medications. Now, I take only two medications at lower doses.

Pete's 5 Fasting Tips:

1. Eat fat-rich foods before you fast - Once fasting begins, sugars are depleted. Fat is the remaining energy source. By lowering basal insulin levels, you utilize fat for energy. Fats stored longer will be burned first.
2. Reduce protein when beginning your fast - In the days prior to fasting, I start reducing protein while gradually increasing fat consumption. I like to add avocados early on, as they seem to promote fat-burning. If have a low fat,

high protein meal, such as white, skinless chicken, I add butter, cheese or extra virgin olive oil.

3. Listen to your body's signaling system - Once I eliminated processed foods, my hormone balance (E.g., insulin/glucagon, leptin/ghrelin) slowly returned to normal. This resulted in eating when hungry and not eating when full. This signaling helps control hunger during a fast.

4. Add fat to your drinks - If extending my fast to meet my goal becomes difficult, I make black coffee or tea "Mock Latte". I like one tablespoon of grass fed butter or MCT oil for these drinks. I use a frother to blend the mixture. In a snap, I have a satisfying beverage.

5. Drink black coffee with salt - I add Himalayan salt to my coffee because it cuts its bitterness and helps the hydration process. If you use a coffee machine with a basket, add some salt as the coffee brews. This trick enhances the flavor of the coffee.

6. Always eat whole foods – It's what we were intended to eat. I like to use organic produce. I avoid typical supermarket meats. I prefer wild-caught and/or grass-fed cuts. Although more expensive, the reduced quantity consumed offsets the additional cost. Now, I can afford to spend more money per pound on better foods.

Autophagy

By Pete Kaye

What is autophagy? Autophagy is a process that recycles damaged cells and prepares others, such as pre-cancerous cells, for programmed destruction through apoptosis. Why is this important?

People who undergo bariatric surgery always lose a lot of weight. What is left is excess skin that must be removed surgically. This "skin" is actually an accumulation of stored proteins that were not utilized for energy. Had these patients elected to fast, autophagy and apoptosis could have been just as effective. By encouraging his patients to fast, Dr. Fung has never referred anyone for excess skin removal surgery.

How does autophagy impact the brain?

Alzheimer's disease is characterized by an abnormal accumulation of proteins in the brain. These proteins are called amyloid plaques, partly responsible for the symptoms of this disease. The combination of autophagy and apoptosis can be helpful prevention or treatment.

When we fast, autophagy and apoptosis begins. When we feed, this process stops. Without this cycle, runaway autophagy could be harmful.

All about Protein

By Pete Kaye

How much protein does the body need? We know carbohydrates raise insulin, especially carbohydrates devoid of their native fiber, such as white sugar. We also know that leaner proteins also cause an insulin response.

Fact: Dr. Fung has never endorsed counting macros because it's too complicated to explain to his patients. For those who are not intimidated by the math, it can be good exercise to know how much you're actually eating. There are several online apps available to log your food and track your macros.

Many sources use different formulas to calculate protein intake, but Dr. Fung suggests 0.6 grams per kilogram of ideal body weight, which is what I use.

The easiest way to calculate this is to take your ideal body weight in kilograms and have roughly one gram of protein per kilogram, minus 10%. If you have an especially active lifestyle, you can add 5-10 grams more. Men may consume more.

Remember, this is 15 grams of <u>protein</u>, not 15 grams of meat. The meat will weigh much more as it's also comprised of water and fat.

This calculation doesn't have to be exact, but it's a good ballpark figure to keep in mind when you're eating.

Ketogenic Diets

By Gina More Minis

Gina's before and after:

Before: In 2012, my weight was nearly 300 lbs. Weight loss was not considered until I realized my blood glucose was 220. I had high blood pressure and high triglycerides. I had debilitating migraines and experienced severe, body-wide pain, to the point of requiring the use of a cane and becoming home-bound.

After: As of this writing, I have lost 180 lbs. My A1C went from 5.8 to 4.9. My fasting insulin dropped to 1.2. My CRP dropped to 0.1. The migraines and pain are gone. I don't need a cane and can walk up to 6 miles per day.

Most people transition from a low carbohydrate diet to a low carbohydrate, high fat (LCHF) diet and ultimately choose a ketogenic diet. What is a ketogenic diet, though, and how does it differ from LCHF?

The Basics

A ketogenic diet is one of very low carbohydrates (up to 20 grams, from above-ground vegetables), moderate protein (enough to preserve muscle mass) and high fat (where most of your calories will come from). The dietary distribution of calories should consist of 10% or less of carbohydrates, 20% of protein and 70% or more of fat. Protein is eaten in moderation or in accordance to activity level and body composition. The diet does not count calories.

Ketogenic diets starve the body of sugar and force it to use fat as its primary source of fuel. It does this through the use of ketone bodies. Because of the very low carbohydrate allowance, the diet is different than a standard LCHF diet which allows carbohydrates to go up to 30 grams. There are also some low carbohydrate diets that do not put a restriction on protein.

Protein triggers an insulin response and therefore is restricted. Insulin inhibits the action of ketones and fat-burning. The whole purpose of a ketogenic diet is to draw fuel from ketones. This is done by maintaining low insulin levels. So in essence, the diet is aiming to utilize stored fat for fuel without new fat build-up. It is restarting the body's ability to easily shift from glucose to fat, and visa-versa, for energy.

Are There Risks?

If you are relatively healthy, this diet is healthy, if done correctly.

A ketogenic diet is a metabolic therapy, not simply a weight loss diet. It is changing your metabolism to primarily depend on fat for fuel. As a result, glucose and insulin levels drop significantly.

This can cause adverse effects for people who have pre-existing medical conditions, such as diabetes, especially while on glucose-lowering medications. This is why you should first consult your doctor before starting this type of therapeutic diet.

Is It For Everyone?

Ketogenic diets are for everyone. In fact, they have been around for 99% of human existence. We survived and thrived because carbohydrates were not around all the time, especially during ice ages. Our metabolism therefore evolved to utilize ketones. This diet allows us to revive this ability.

Fact: Any metabolic change causes hormonal stress. When you gain a lot of weight, your hormones become imbalanced. This is why obese women, or women who gain weight, tend to lose their menstrual cycles. The same applies for weight loss. It can take several months for your hormone balance to adjust to your new size and body composition. Over time, homeostasis is achieved.

It's important to keep in mind the adverse effects observed in some people, which are not caused by the ketogenic diet itself, rather by its improper implementation and/or dependence of glucose for energy. The abnormalities observed are actually caused by prolonged, excessive carbohydrate consumption, which trigger hypoglycemia while on ketosis.

Is There Only One Way To Be Ketogenic?

No. There are various versions of ketogenic diets. Each has a different set of macro-nutrient allowances. Your choice depends on goals.

You can apply a ketogenic, macro-nutrient profile to any diet, for example, the vegetarian ketogenic diet.

Some ketogenic diets restrict carbohydrates and/or protein more than others. Carbohydrate ranges are 10g to 50g per day. Some people reap the benefits of mild ketosis just as much as those in full ketosis.

Ketone Testing

How do you know if you are in ketosis?

If you have low fasting insulin levels, stable blood glucose levels and can endure more than 12 hours of water fasting, then you are reaping the benefits of nutritional ketosis. Testing is not required.

There are several products available to test for the presence of ketones. These include ketone urine test strips, ketone breathalyzers and blood ketone meters. All of these work differently and are a topic for debate. Just because ketones are present, does not mean they are being utilized, especially with elevated insulin levels.

People that are following a ketogenic diet for the treatment of seizure disorders, cancer or other medical conditions are under medical supervision and their doctor should be measuring their ketone levels.

Exogenous Ketones

Exogenous ketones are not required for nutritional ketosis.

People that need to follow a ketogenic diet for the treatment of serious medical conditions, such as cancer, neurodegenerative disorders or seizures are often given exogenous ketones by their doctors. These exogenous ketones are often required under these circumstances.

When following a ketogenic diet for metabolic health and weight loss, you want your body to produce and utilize its own ketones. This ensures that insulin is low when ketones are high. Any other variation will cause ketones to be converted to fat instead of being used for fuel.

Fact: The elusive "keto rash" is a mildly itchy rash many people develop after going into ketosis. The rash usually occurs on the back and trunk, but can affect extremities as well. There have been many theories as to the cause, but the consensus seems to be ketones themselves are the culprit. Ketones contain acetone, which can be irritating in high concentrations. Applying raw apple cider vinegar, coconut oil or cocoa butter to the rash is beneficial.

Ketogenic Products

The best aspect of ketogenic diets also applies to fasting. It's FREE! Remember, this diet is based on REAL food.

So, no matter what anyone claims, there is no such thing as a "keto" snack. People on compliant ketogenic diets, do not consume "keto"-branded products in the form of supplements, bars, drinks, powders, etc. These are by default not ketogenic.

Fat Adaptation

Fat adaptation or to be "fat adapted" means your body can now rely on dietary fat for fuel versus glucose. In other words, your insulin levels have dropped enough to use and not store fat for fuel.

You do not have to be fat adapted to lose weight. We know this because people on low fat diets also lose weight. Fat adaptation simply changes your metabolism to use fat as its primary fuel, and switch to glucose only through gluconeogenesis. Glucose is not a primary source of fuel anymore.

If you are fat adapted, you are able to fast for longer than 12 hours without fatigue, weakness, hunger, exhaustion, dizziness and/or inappropriate blood glucose fluctuations.

Counting Macros

There are many online tools that will help you log your food and track your macro-nutrients.

There is no wrong way to calculate macro-nutrients. You can count the grams per meal or per day or focus on the daily caloric composition percentages. I prefer to use percentages because I do not count calories.

If nutritional ketosis is what you're aiming for, then the easiest approach is to have up to three meals per day, without snacking in between. Just remember to:

- Eat to satiety, without counting calories
- Do not snack
- Do not avoid fat or purposely over-consume it to reach its percentage goal
- Reduce carbohydrates to only above-ground vegetables

Remember, ketogenic diets are not about eating excessive butter or frying bacon in coconut oil. You simply choose foods with their natural macro-nutrients intact. Do not consume anything that is marked as fat free, low fat, reduced fat or cholesterol free.

Fact: Leptin resistance accompanies insulin resistance in obesity. When you are leptin resistant, your metabolism does not accelerate and your appetite does not decrease, even with added dietary fat. The extra fat is stored and your body does not respond to leptin signaling for satiety. Therefore, you do not achieve weight loss benefits. Eat whole foods containing full fat at mealtimes and avoid snacks.

How To Start

To begin a ketogenic diet, you don't do so abruptly. You slowly acclimate to it.

- Remove all sugars and grains first, followed by starches. Then incorporate fat-rich foods

- Stop all snacking. Consume no more than 3 meals per day. This will give you a 16-18 hour fasting period and lower insulin levels to allow your body to draw fuel from fat stores
- Take a magnesium supplement (400 IU per day)
- Stay well hydrated
- Generously salt your food with Himalayan salt to help maintain healthy electrolyte balance

A ketogenic diet will simplify your fasting protocol and provide your metabolism the flexibility to primarily use fat for fuel and endogenous glucose as necessary. This will free you from the shackles of exogenous sugar.

Why Gina Fasts:

1. To prevent Alzheimer's and cancer
2. To treat seizures
3. To treat migraines with aura
4. To maintain weight loss
5. To improve insulin sensitivity
6. To find homeostasis

Gina's 4 Fasting Tips:

1. Fast according to your circadian rhythm: Proper timing helps you reach your goals. I prefer fasting during the afternoons. That is when I am least hungry and most active.
2. Eat to fast: Eat a satisfying, fatty meal before fasting.
3. Fast away from home: I like to fast while running errands or exercising. It avoids poor food choices found away from home.
4. Avoid high carbohydrate meals: This will prevent your liver from storing excess glycogen, to be released while fasting. This release of glycogen is akin to consuming sugar while you are trying to fast. Therefore, avoiding excess glycogen stores will allow them to be depleted quickly while fasting. As a result, you will be able to tap into your fat stores for fuel and induce autophagy, providing the maximum benefits from your fast.

What about Cholesterol?

By Gina More Minis

There is still a lot to know about cholesterol and what its effects are in the context of a low carb, high fat diet. This has not been studied enough yet.

I can only tell you my experience. I have a cholesterol of 420. I am Pattern A (low risk for heart disease). I have been on a high fat, low carb diet for several years, and my cholesterol has lowered slowly.

Before I went on a high fat diet, my cholesterol was always in the mid 200's. Trying to control my cholesterol with a low fat diet nearly gave me diabetes. It is known that diabetes puts me at a high risk for heart disease. High cholesterol, however, has not been proven to do so. Therefore, I'll take my chances with the unknown or not yet proven. If I drop dead in a few years, I at least avoided a wheelchair, dialysis, loss of vision and limbs.

Cholesterol usually comes up in discussions about low carb, high fat diets. After all, it is the reason I believe the erroneous dietary guidelines were created.

Fact: Common lipid panels will flag a High Total Cholesterol as "high risk". These panels use the Total Cholesterol to HDL ratio to determine risk. That ratio categorizes large groups of people as "high risk", and as candidates for statin drugs. The most predictive ratio is your Triglycerides to HDL, which is directly linked to cardiac outcomes. The reference values should be: 5 or less = good, 3 or less = best, 1 or less = optimal.

Here are some current facts about cholesterol, which might motivate you to do more research before deciding to interpret your numbers.

Total Cholesterol Number Facts:

- There is no upper limit to cholesterol because it is benign. The Total Cholesterol number your doctor classifies as "normal" or "abnormal" fails to provide useful information. No study has ever proven that this number accurately predicts cardiac disease risk. In fact, the only correlation found between cholesterol and disease risk is Low HDL.

- Eating saturated fats increases LDL Cholesterol for some, and significantly for a rare few. These people are considered "hyper-responders", who are in essence not likelier to increase their cardiac risk because a high LDL count, on its own, is meaningless.

- The reason people get heart attacks, regardless of their cholesterol levels, is that heart disease has everything to do with oxidative stress (damage), which leads to inflammation. This is why diabetics are at such a high risk for heart disease. Diabetes is a disease of very high oxidation.

- Your Total Cholesterol doesn't matter because it doesn't measure the degree of lipoprotein oxidation. Knowing your particle size and density provides more useful, yet incomplete information. This is because large, buoyant particles tend to be less oxidized than small, dense particles, yet people with large, buoyant particles also suffer from heart attacks. This is because what you really want to know is how oxidized your lipoprotein particles are.

Best Tests to Have If You're Worried About Cholesterol:

- Advanced Lipid Panel: Measures cholesterol particle size. Aim for Pattern A
- Oxidized LDL Panel – Similar to A1C, it shows you how at risk you are for metabolic syndrome by measuring the oxidation of your LDL particles. Aim for less than 60, which puts you at low risk.
- Omega 3 to Omega 6 Ratio – It measures how much Omega 3 or Omega 6 fatty acids you are consuming. Aim for a ratio of 1:1 in favor of Omega 3 fatty acids.
- Triglycerides and HDL - Triglycerides should be less than 100 and HDL should be over 60.
- Highly Sensitive C-Reactive protein - This is a blood test marker for inflammation, and should be less than < 1.0 mg/L.

What to Do About It:

Elevated LDL increases the risk of oxidation. It is not predictive of heart disease. Only its oxidation is predictive. So, a very high LDL number on a high oxidative diet is completely different than a high LDL number on a low oxidative diet.

The best thing you can do to protect LDL from oxidation is to restrict carbohydrates. Carbohydrates or sugar as fuel causes oxidation. If you're a fat burner, you've opted for a cleaner fuel to protect your LDL. Whereas a high carbohydrate diet promotes metabolic abnormalities that eventually lead to metabolic syndrome.

Metabolic syndrome promotes malignancy within the body, primarily chronic systemic inflammation. It is, therefore, the number one risk factor for developing heart disease. This is why the American Heart Association (AHA) has failed to prevent a single heart attack since its recommendation and endorsement of "heart-healthy" carbohydrates for those of us with high cholesterol. The AHA is actually killing you faster.

Fact: Total cholesterol was never a diagnostic marker of metabolic syndrome because no correlation has ever been found between the two. Currently, the American Diabetes Association has decided to consider it a marker in the wake of a thriving statin market. The only markers that have ever been used to determine metabolic dysfunction on a lipid panel is low HDL and high triglycerides.

- Avoid seed oils. These "heart-healthy" seed oils are highly oxidized and unstable. They will damage your lipids just like carbohydrates ("sugar") will.
- Choose a low carbohydrate diet. This allows your insulin to remain low. High insulin leads to endothelial dysfunction, arterial plaque and blood clots.
- Choose healthy fats. Although coconut oil is healthy, if your LDL is very high, ease off the coconut oil. Its lauric acid has the tendency to make hyper-responders into ultra-responders. Instead, choose butter or ghee and increase your mono-unsaturated fats with avocado, macadamia or olive oils.

- Fast. Intermittent fasting is beneficial because the body is forced to utilize the fat circulating in the blood as fuel while helping manage oxidative stress. Digestion causes a lot of oxidation while fasting has the opposite effect. So it makes sense to fast.

Fact: *The term "familial hypercholesterolemia" is mentioned in your doctor's office even though only a lipid specialist can diagnose this genetic condition with genetic testing. Total Cholesterol is not diagnostic. Even though there are two genetic pathways for hypercholesterolemia, there are actually many different manifestations. Lipid abnormalities are so numerous and rare that little is known about them. Some who have tested positive for lipid abnormalities do not reveal any active disease process.*

To Snack or Not To Snack

By Gina More Minis

Snacking keeps insulin elevated for extended periods, unlike how it's supposed to work. Insulin is released in pulses. This means that it increases when you eat and decreases when you don't. The body does this to avoid resistance. There are three incretin pathways for insulin. Snacking stimulates all of them all the time.

The calories of the snack make no difference. The macro-nutrients of the snack make no difference. There is no "good" snack. There is no "healthy" snack.

If you like cheese and nuts, incorporate them into your meals and avoid them as snacks. As low-carb "snacks", they are very unhealthy. Any food that is used as a snack is unhealthy, even kale.

Eat your meals at meal times only.

Fact: If you are bored and want to snack, find other activities to do. These include reading, gardening, cleaning, organizing, walking, window shopping, calling a friend, solving crossword puzzles and playing computer games.

But what about coffee?

Do not snack on bullet-proof coffee (BPC). A lot of people believe BPC gets a pass because of its high fat content - not so fast.

Bullet proof coffee is a very high fat drink introduced to new followers to help them become fat adapted and prepare for fasting. It is usually made with 8-12 ounces of coffee, 1 tsp. - 2 tbsp. of MCT oil, butter or ghee, blended together.

Here are two correct ways to use bullet-proof coffee:

1. You've just begun the low carb, high fat diet and are learning how to add fats to your meals. You choose BPC instead of your typical high carbohydrate breakfast.

Your cup of BPC will get you through the morning, energized and without the usual mid-day hypoglycemic crash. You found you were able to skip lunch and eat dinner instead.

2. You are planning an extended fast, so you start with a fat fast. You decide to drink a BPC for breakfast, followed by a bacon, avocado and olive meal for lunch, to become fat adapted. You drink another BPC for dinner. Now, you are able to start your weekend fast with plenty of fat for fuel.

BPC can be the only "meal" of the day for an extended fast.

As you can see, in both of these scenarios, the BPC was used to *replace* a meal.

Some people drink BPC as a snack between meals or to accompany a high fat meal. This will cause weight gain or stalling.

You cannot snack on BPC or heavy whipping cream coffees and expect weight-loss to continue. A high fat meal does not give you a pass to "eat whatever you want, whenever you want it". Doing so will be just as detrimental as the carbohydrates were. You are eating all of the time and filling your cells with fat instead of sugar! The same behavior will get you the same results.

The Perils of Sweeteners

By Gina More Minis

People always ask about artificial sweeteners and the answer is that using them will not be beneficial to your new lifestyle. Here are some reasons why.

1. They're artificial. This fact should be enough to exclude them from your diet. Diets used to treat metabolic diseases are based on natural, whole foods. Artificial sweeteners do not fall into this category. They are the industry's latest attempt to overcome an ever-increasing epidemic caused by their "unhealthy foods".

2. There is no such thing as a "natural" artificial sweetener. Those two words cannot be used in the same sentence. Stevia is not found in nature as a white powder. It is a green leaf from a plant. Indigenous people have never used this leaf to bake "low carb" cakes and pies. In short, even if the source is natural or wholesome, once it has been processed or changed, it is no longer natural.

Fact: Stevia does not raise insulin levels at the 30 or 60 minutes mark, after consumption, but it increases it astronomically at the 120 minutes mark. This means that if you thought you were fasting while adding Stevia to your drinks, think again.

3. You cannot "trick" the human body. You cannot trick a system that has been evolving way before you were born. It will respond to environmental and digestive cues and modify its response to remain in homeostasis, even if that change results in metabolic derangement initiated by the host. Simply speaking, there is no such thing as a "no calorie" and "sweet" food on planet earth.

4. Most sweeteners are primarily used in drinks. The body did not evolve to drink its calories. That's why water has 0 calories and is flavorless. It does not trigger a digestive response or release of hormones. Artificial sweeteners trigger false alarms of incoming energy that never arrives. This is a recipe for metabolic chaos.

5. Consumption of sweeteners sabotage your goals. If you are seeking to incorporate or continue eating certain foods of the Standard American Diet (SAD) diet, then you are not ready to make a lifestyle change. Those food choices cannot exist while on a ketogenic or low carbohydrate diet. Sweeteners will inevitably lure you back to poor health and obesity. It's time for something new.

6. All sweeteners, including artificial ones, have been shown to raise insulin levels. Metabolic disease is a disease of hormones, primarily insulin. If you are still stimulating your insulin levels while having 0 calories and unchanged blood glucose, you have failed to improve your health.

7. Artificial sweeteners have failed to halt metabolic disease progression. Since introduced, artificial sweeteners have not prevented weight gain and diabetes. In fact, obesity and diabetes are at an all-time high. How sweeteners perpetuate obesity has been debated for years, but a growing consensus is that they are not the solution. If they aren't part of the solution, they can only be part of the problem.

Fact: Artificial sweeteners are bad; "natural" sugar is no better. Honey, maple syrup, agave nectar and coconut sugar, for example, are sugars. If you are sick and consume them, you will get sicker. If you are healthy and consume them, you will become sick like everyone else. The path to diabetes can take multiple routes. Consuming sugar, in all of its forms, will adversely affect your health. Our bodies do not like exogenous sugar. It likes to create and use its own glucose, as needed.

---

8. Artificial sweeteners are mainly used by diabetics to bake cakes, but at what cost? There is always give and take. We already know what happens when you want your cake and eat it too. Insulin injections become necessary. This mindset won't lead to improvement of health. Avoiding sweet foods is a good way to secure a healthy prognosis.

Weight Stalling

By Gina More Minis

What can cause a weight stall?

Stalling during weight loss is normal. The body loses weight and then reconfigures itself around the lost weight. This takes time. It has to rearrange blood vessels, connective tissue, protein, collagen, etc. Generally, the body will lose weight for a while and then go through this process of reconfiguring where it halts weight loss. This is a "stall" or "plateau", where the body is just catching up and adapting to its own weight loss and new composition. But, these stalls should not be prolonged.

It is hard to determine how long they should be because it all depends on how much weight is being lost and at what rate. Generally, a stall starts becoming suspicious when it lasts more than 3 months. That's when it's time to do something about it. Many people will be faced with this problem. Everyone is different, so the reasons can be multifaceted. I will list some common mistakes that can be contributing to this frustrating situation. Each one of these things affects hormones.

So, before you give up on your new lifestyle, determine if any of these apply to you, change them and monitor progress. This only pertains to those affected by weight stalling. If you are still losing weight, then continue doing whatever you're doing. If it's not broken, don't fix it.

1. Natural Or Artificial Sweeteners.

Until you get rid of ALL sweeteners, you really won't know what's causing your weight stalling or weight gain.

2. Hidden Sugars. A lot of times we buy LCHF items for our meals and neglect to check the ingredients. Checking both ingredients and carb content is vital for making smart food choices.

The carb count only tells you how many carbs there are in a serving. If you decide to eat more than a serving or are consuming this same item regularly, the sugars in it, no matter how trivial, begin adding up. Before you know it, you just ate the equivalent of a candy bar in the form of bacon.

3. Cheating. Cheaters never win. There should be no reason to cheat.

"Cheat days" start adding up. Once you add one, they start multiplying, like bunnies but not as cute. If you're still lamenting your old life, then there is something wrong with your new one and you have to change it.

You must tailor this lifestyle in a way that allows you to follow it consistently by choosing an ancestral diet you enjoy and a fasting regimen you can sustain.

Fact: Fiber slows down the absorption of sugar, but it doesn't eliminate it. This slowdown is actually worse because it will keep your insulin higher, for a longer period of time, as glucose slowly keeps leaking out of your gut into the already overloaded cells that do not want any more glucose. That is why brown rice, quinoa, fruit and "healthy whole grains" have been ineffective in the battle against "diabesity". In fact, the most obese are the biggest consumers of these "healthy foods". The body doesn't care if your blood sugar rises slowly or quickly. The blood sugar is still rising and that's what you need to avoid, so that insulin does not follow suit.

---

4. Snacking. Eat at meal times ONLY and not before, after or between.

Snacking causes a lot of issues. Besides stimulating insulin all of the time, snacking causes people who are leptin resistant to eat too much fat. Snacking often opens the avenue for consuming food in ways we did not evolve to do so, like drinking them. A lot of snacks are "drinks" and drinking your calories has a negative effect on metabolism.

5. Not Eating Enough. You would be surprised how often this happens and how under recognized it is because it's so counterintuitive to what we have been told all of our lives. Here are a couple of behaviors that cause people to not eat enough:

- **Micro-managing and over thinking macros.** Some people stop listening to their bodies and start following a macro app calculator on their phones instead.

- **Over-counting carbs.** Some people are trying to calculate the carbs in an avocado or in green beans.
- **Over eating fat and over restriction of protein.** People are dumping sticks of butter into their food or eating a minute amount of protein a week, just to see ketone levels rise.
- **Portion controlling.** People are serving themselves very small portions and calling these h'orderves a "meal".

There is a fine line between these behaviors and calorie restriction. When that line is crossed, your body will let you know by stalling.

Don't be scared to eat. Eat until you feel satisfied and your stomach extended. Eat real food and don't avoid fat. Don't add fat to meals just to meet a certain macro quota. Your feeding time is very important because you're feeding to fast.

If you don't feel hungry for a large meal, eat in intervals, for a limited period of time. Give yourself a four to six hour feeding window and allow yourself to eat as much as you want during that time. Do not count calories or control portions.

6. Fasting Too Much. You have to balance feeding with fasting.

You cannot feed all of the time or fast all of the time. This is especially true if you are already following a ketogenic diet. These diets mimic the effects of fasting on the body, so you are not required to fast for extended periods. If the fasting is out of balance, the body loses homeostasis.

If you have been on extended fasts for a long time and are not seeing results, try shorter, more frequent fasts instead.

7. Being Too Sedentary. Obesity is hormonal, not caloric. Burning calories through exercise will not make you lose weight, but exercise does affect you hormonally.

Just like you can't eat all of the time or fast all of the time, you certainly cannot sit all of the time. The body needs to be in homeostasis. That is its preferred state. You must balance rest with stress. Exercise puts the body in a mild state of stress that causes it to release hormones that promote development, growth and repair.

When you exercise, you lower insulin and increase the counter regulatory hormones that help mediate insulin's effects. All hormones work in pulses. Exercise is the cue for stress hormones to be released. Rest is the cue for them to be low. Releasing these stress hormones in pulses will make them less likely to be high or low when they shouldn't be. They will be more sensitive to cues rather than resistant to them.

Exercise also burns stored glycogen in the liver and glucose in the muscles. It helps mobilize fat through fatty acid oxidation. It changes your body composition by improving muscle to fat ratio, which contributes to better metabolic health. All of these things help regulate hormonal balance.

Your exercise routine does not have to be strenuous or prolonged. Choose a routine that fits your schedule and lifestyle. Most importantly, choose one that you like. Enjoying your exercise will allow you to remain consistent.

8. Meal Timings. When you eat is as important as what you eat. Switch your meal timings.

If you are eating 2 meals a day, try to eat them earlier in the day. Dr. Fung recommends 10 am – 2 pm as the best eating times.

If you have been doing OMAD (one meal a day) for an extended period of time, you most likely slowed your metabolism. Add more meals to your day, up to three, with no snacking in between.

9. Food Quality. The focus should be on nutrient-dense food with all macros present. This is how food is found in nature. These are the common mistakes people make with their diet:

- **Use of meal replacements.** A lot of people use meal replacement bars and shakes. These processed foods throw your macros out of line. The shakes are especially harmful because they are usually filled with too much and the wrong kind of protein.

  You are also drinking your calories by consuming them, which is never a good idea.

- **Eating junk, "keto style".** Meals should not consist of recipes for "low carb biscuits", "fat bombs" and "keto pancakes". These are considered processed meals – a no, no.

Also, do not fall prey to those selling "low carb, high fat" junk food. These people are no better than Big Food selling "low fat/low calorie" junk food. Eat real food, with all of the macro-nutrients they naturally contain.

- **Recipe cards – no end in sight.** Do not rely solely on elaborate "recipes". Stick with simple ones, and as you become more familiar with your diet and how it impacts you, you may incorporate them. Start with the basics.

Low carb, high fat needs no recipes because there is no baking involved. It's just meat and vegetables.

Cook your favorite meat and vegetables, in your favorite way, using healthy, natural fats. Cold salads take very little preparation time. Healthy ingredients, like olives, nuts, avocados, cheeses, etc., can be added to them. All the goodies you wish to snack on can be a salad topping for one of your meals.

10. The Wrong Definition of Feasting. When you are feasting, it should not be at a fast food restaurant.

You should be eating nutrient-dense, real food in accordance to a healthy metabolic profile, which is low carb, high fat. People give this "feasting" an entirely inappropriate meaning and start feasting on pies and cakes.

If you use your feeding times to eat junk food, you will fill your glycogen stores to capacity and basically, you will be eating that stored glucose during your fast. This means that you're never truly fasting, even though you're not eating. Your liver has become a chocolate cake buffet that you're feeding on during your fasting hours.

11. Shake Up Your Macros. This can shake up metabolism and is especially needed if you track macros very closely, and have been doing so for a long time.

If you have been consistently on a ketogenic diet, eating the recommended macros and implementing intermittent fasting, but yet your weight has stalled, switch up your macros. You might have to increase protein intake and/or carbohydrate levels with squashes and tubers, for example.

Cycling in and out of ketosis, even on a "lazy keto" diet, can be a very powerful tool for some. On a "lazy keto" diet, you are not strictly tracking your macros. This allows a higher amount of protein or carbohydrates in the diet to enter a mildly ketotic state versus high ketotic state. Some people thrive in mild ketosis and not so much in full ketosis.

11. Change Your Diet. Do not let dogma keep you in a stalled state. Your goal is to improve your health and lose weight. If the diet you are on, ketogenic or otherwise, is not getting you there - change it.

I know there are many who want to hold on to their beloved diet and the belief that it HAS to work, but "the proof is in the pudding", as Dr. Fung has said. If it truly worked, then it would be working. If it isn't, it's time for it to go the way of the dinosaurs.

Choose an ancestral diet that fits with your lifestyle and preference. By ancestral diet, I mean a REAL FOOD diet. None of the following is permitted: sugar/sweeteners, grains, processed foods, calorie counting, low fat, drinking calories and controlling portions. (In every case, consuming grains is not an option with metabolic dysfunction, so remove them from your diet and replace them with vegetables instead.)

12. Other Things to Consider:

Keep in mind that certain medications can create weight gain or weight stalling. This is where diet can make all of the difference since prescription medications must be continued.

If medications, like synthetic cortisol, release too much glucose from the cells and keeps insulin levels high all of the time, then avoiding exogenous sugar will help tremendously. If you do not consume exogenous sugar, then cortisol will dump out less glucose from the cells.

If you suspect your medications are causing an issue with your weight, discuss this with your doctor. If your doctor can explain HOW the medication causes the weight gain, you will be able to find dietary avenues to mitigate these effects.

Testimonials

By Fung Shweigh Group Members

From Sarah-Louise Moseley

I've struggled with my weight for years. I've tried all kinds of plans while my checkbook balance got smaller. When I found Dr. Fung's, "The Obesity Code" book, it was a light bulb moment for me. Everything suddenly made sense. I was fortunate enough to come across the Fung Shweigh Facebook Group at the start of my journey and the support has been immeasurable. I'm no longer held hostage by hunger and cravings and can complete 5 day fasts with ease and peace of mind. The Fasting Fungsters Recipe Group has been a safe haven for me, providing a variety of healthy recipe choices for me to choose from. After 8 months, I've lost just over 235 lbs., improved my fitness and corrected numerous health issues. Thank you Dr. Fung & the Fung Shweigh team.

"I want people to realize that it's not a quick or linear journey, but if you stick with it, you will see improvement." – Denise Arneson's

From Jeri Labell

I am honored to share my story. On May of 2016, I was at the cardiologist, welcomed by my 25 years of diabetic complications and insulin toxicity. After 15 years, insulin increased to 80 units a day. I had developed heart failure, obesity, diabetic autonomic neuropathy that causes gastro-paresis, where food does not move along the digestive tract as it should. It caused constipation and vomiting. I felt like I was dying. I needed to make the choice of life or death. I am the one who puts the fork in my mouth, so the choice is mine. I decided to join the Intensive Dietary Management Program. Since then, I have lost over 60 lbs from 225 lbs. I was able to get off the insulin at age 60. Doing intermittent fasting and the low carb, high fat diet is my new way of life. Now, I am off ALL medications and have significantly improved health by 95% I thank GOD for Dr. Fung and Megan Ramos.

From Joshua Clark

I received The Complete Guide to Fasting, as a gift from Sandy T. Rodriguez, about a month ago. I started cutting out carbs and other processed foods. I have also done some intermittent fasting. I really was only interested in controlling my blood glucose, which was at the 120-130 range at that time. In a month, I have lost 15 lbs., and blood glucose dropped to 105. Thanks for all your research and hard work, Dr. Fung!

"As food quantity decreases, quality of life increases." – Gina More Minis.

From Manny Gomez

When I was first diagnosed with type 2 diabetes, it seemed like the cherry on top of a bad health Sunday. I was obviously severely obese, but was not connecting the dots as to how that related to other health issues, like blurry vision, excruciating morning foot pain and waking up choking in the middle of the night. Now, I had a prolonged, slow, death sentence, filled with poking myself with needles and drugs. Doing the same failed things repeatedly was not an option anymore. Luckily, the internet led me to Dr. Fung. It was life-changing. Luckily, Facebook has the largest online group that adheres to Dr. Fung's life-saving protocol: Fung Shweigh.

From Denise Arneson

Two and a half years ago, I was diagnosed with type 2 diabetes. I found a Facebook group that used the low carb, high fat diet to achieve blood glucose control. My blood sugar got better and I lost weight, but then I stalled out. The group I joined mentioned Dr. Fung. So, I Googled him and read every blog entry that he ever wrote. I started eating in a 6-8 hour window and doing longer fasts. Low carb, high fat wasn't enough for me to achieve normal blood glucose. I needed to fast because my insulin was too high. I started with an A1C of 7.3 and today my A1C is 5.2 which is in normal range. I've also lost 80 lbs., and have kept it off. More improvement is needed, but with enough time and fasting I will achieve my goals.

From Moneca Avgm

I have been struggling with obesity my whole life. I have tried many diets, products, doctors and books. My first diet was at age 7. Doctors, family, friends and media gave me the same advice: it is a matter of balance between calories in and calories out. Restrict caloric intake and exercise more. I would lose weight and gain it back. Then another new diet, new doctor, new goal. I was sure it wasn't my fault. Everyone said it was. "It is a matter of willpower. Maybe you haven't tried enough". I knew it wasn't true, but I couldn't prove my belief to regain self-esteem.

In April 2016, when I was 43 years old, 255 lbs., pre-diabetic and suffering from high blood pressure and fatty liver, I discovered Dr. Fung's "Obesity Code" book. Someone from Canada and far away from Spain, where I live, gave me all the answers I was looking for all my life. Suddenly everything made sense for me. It wasn't my fault and a solution was at hand, cheap and straightforward. I started the LCHF dietary protocol July 21st with 24 hours of intermittent fasting every day. In October, I joined the IDM program with noticeable improvements. I was able to complete extended fasts of up to 3 days. Eventually, glucose, HbA1c, fasting insulin, CRP and other inflammatory markers (as ESR) returned to a normal range. 10 months later, I lost 100lbs, reversed fatty liver disease and got off my high blood pressure medication. I have more energy than ever before. I have no cravings, migraines and weakness anymore. It was my willpower and the correct protocol that helped me so much. My doctors still think I am crazy when I speak of LCHF and fasting, but I don't care!

Recipes

Simple Meatless Wrap Fajita Style by Sandy Tucker Rodriguez:

- 4 Portobello mushrooms (brown gills scraped off), sliced
- ½ large green bell pepper, sliced
- ½ red bell pepper, sliced
- 2 jalapeno chili peppers, minced (to taste or use salsa)
- 1 large onion, sliced
- 1 handful of chopped cilantro
- 8 oz. shredded cheese to garnish (I like pepper jack)
- 4 romaine lettuce leaves
- Ghee, butter, lard or other fat of your choosing
- Salt and pepper to taste

Add 2 tbsp. of chosen fat to hot skillet. Add sliced mushrooms and dry about 8-10 mins until tender.

Add peppers and onion, cook for 2-3 mins more.

Season and add salsa or jalapenos (if using) and cilantro now. Simmer 1 min more.

Toss all to mix flavors. Divide mixture into the lettuce leaves and add cheese to top. Roll like a burrito.

Easy Guacamole by Sandy Tucker Rodriguez:

- 2 ripe avocados
- About ¼ cup onion, minced
- 1-2 chilies, with stems and seeds removed, minced (your choice to omit)
- 2 tbsp. cilantro leaves, chopped
- 1 tbsp. fresh lime juice
- ½ ripe tomato, chopped
- Salt and pepper to taste

Cut avocados in half, remove large pit and scoop out avocado from the peel. Place in a mixing bowl.

Using a fork, mash the avocado and add the chopped onion, cilantro, lime and seasoning. Mash some more to incorporate ingredients. Now add your chili pepper, if you like.

Mix in tomatoes last so they aren't smashed. Eat right away as guacamole will turn dark in color when exposed to air too long. Serve with vegetable sticks.

Helpful hint: Be careful when handling peppers so you do not irritate your eyes.

Sandy's Favorite Foods:
Fats: butter, extra virgin olive oil, heavy cream, coconut oil
Protein: Bacon, salmon, tuna, pork belly
Nuts/Seeds: macadamias, almonds, pecans, walnuts, sunflower seeds
Vegetables: Romaine, radish, cucumber, celery, cabbage, spinach, green beans, onions
Fruit: Raspberries, strawberries, avocado, olives

Easy Cream of Broccoli Soup by Sandy Tucker Rodriguez:

- 3-4 cups fresh broccoli
- 2 tbsp. butter
- 1 cup water or fresh chicken broth (canned can be used too)
- 1 clove garlic
- 1 tbsp. onion, minced
- 1 cup heavy cream
- Parmesan cheese (optional)
- Salt and pepper to taste

Cook broccoli in water until well done. In another large pot, add butter, broth, garlic, onion and seasonings. Then add cooked broccoli.

Cook and stir until the broccoli falls apart, (mash a little if needed).

Add heavy cream and gently bring to a boil. Cook until mixed and creamy.

Sprinkle parmesan cheese, if desired.

Fried Radishes by Sandy Tucker Rodriguez:

- 1 bunch of red radishes cleaned and chopped
- 2 green onions chopped
- 1/2 green bell pepper chopped
- Salt and pepper to taste
- 1 Tb. coconut oil

Heat oil and add chopped radishes.

Cook for 5 min, then add remaining vegetables. Cook until tender and season.

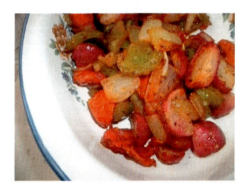

BLT in A Bowl by Sandy Tucker Rodriguez:

- 1 large head of lettuce, torn
- 1 pint of cherry tomatoes, halved
- ½ small red onion, chopped
- ½ lb. bacon, cooked and crumbled
- Salt and pepper to taste

Cook bacon first and save the warm bacon fat. Place torn lettuce in a large bowl.

Layer halved tomatoes on lettuce, then sprinkle on chopped onions and seasoning. Place crumbled bacon on top.

Use the warm bacon drippings to pour over the salad as a dressing, to wilt the lettuce, or you can use your favorite dressing if desired.

Salmon Patties by Sandy Tucker Rodriguez:

- 6 oz. can salmon, drained
- ½ small onion, diced
- ¼ cup Parmesan cheese, grated
- 2 eggs, cracked and beaten
- 1 tbsp. olive or coconut oil
- Black pepper to taste

In medium bowl, combine salmon, onion, parmesan cheese, eggs and black pepper.

Mix well and form into patties.

In a nonstick frying pan, fry patties in olive or coconut oil until browned on both sides.

Low Carb "Universal" Breading by Pete Kaye:

This recipe works for veal, pork, and chicken cutlets. These meats can be sliced to a half inch thickness and pounded flat until they are as large and thick as you like them. This recipe will be enough to make one pound of cutlets. I have done this with eggplant and larger zucchini with success.

When I make this recipe, I generally make several pounds at a time. I find it just as easy to clean up after frying 5 pounds as one pound. These cutlets freeze well, so keep that in mind.

- ½ cup coconut flour
- ½ cup ground almond flour
- ½ cup grated Italian cheese (the drier, the better)
- ¼ cup ground flaxseed meal (I try to sneak this into anything I can think of)
- Salt and pepper to taste (the dry mix needs generous seasoning)
- 1 egg plus a tsp. of water beaten into an egg wash
- Oil for frying (Coconut oil is great. My preference is EVOO, at a low heat)

Use three plates to make a dredging station. Plate 1 gets the coconut flour. Plate two gets the egg wash. Plate 3 gets the rest of the dry ingredients, mixed to an even consistency.

Heat the oil for frying. Dredge a cutlet in plate 1, next dip the cutlet into the egg wash. Finally dredge the wet cutlet into the mixture in plate 3. Slowly slide the cutlet into the oil and fry until golden. Drain on a paper towel.

Continue to fry until all the cutlets are done, adding oil as necessary.

These can now be coated with any sauce you like. Parmesan style is a crowd pleaser. I have also used my frying oil as the base for a sauce made by adding some diced onion, garlic, seasonings, deglazing with some wine that I reduce. Then you can add some heavy whipping cream or some cubes of cold butter to finish the sauce. Use your imagination!

Homemade Pork Sausages by Sandy Tucker Rodriguez:

- 1 lb. ground pork
- 1 tbsp. dried sage
- ½ tsp. cumin
- ¼ cup fresh parsley, minced
- ¼ tsp. cayenne pepper or a pinch of red pepper flakes
- ¼ tsp. salt
- 1 tsp. black pepper

Mix all ingredients well and make patties. The patties can be frozen individually until ready to be fried. Wrap them in foil or plastic wrap to freeze.

Depending on the size you make the patties, this recipe will make 8 patties.

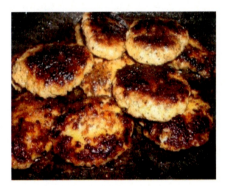

Broccoli and Cheese Patties by Sandy Tucker Rodriguez:

- 1 cup cooked broccoli
- ¼ cup mozzarella cheese, grated
- 1 tbsp. chopped onion
- 1 egg, cracked and beaten
- 1 tsp coconut oil
- Salt and pepper to taste

On a plate, mash the cooked, very soft broccoli with a fork. In a medium bowl, combine mashed broccoli, mozzarella cheese, onion, egg and seasoning. Form tablespoons of mixture.

In a nonstick skillet, add coconut oil and hear over medium heat. Add patties to skillet and cook until brown underneath. Flip over gently and cook on the other side until browned as well.

Helpful hint: Do not flip until the patties are brown around the edges.

Electrolyte Soup by Pete Kaye:

For the vegetarian Fasting Fungsters who cannot eat bone broth, here is a cool idea for a potassium rich, electrolyte rich soup for you.

- Fresh garlic
- 1 large onions, cleaned but with skin left on
- Celery – the base of the celery should be cleaned and chopped
- Kale – chopped, even the ribs are good here
- Potato (peels only provided you have another use for the potato meat)
- As much jarred pepperoncini as you like (I use some of the vinegary juice as well)
- Frozen spinach (one of the best bargains you'll find in the entire supermarket)
- Dandelion greens, or other dark leafy greens
- Mushrooms (you pick the type)
- Eggplant (I use the eggplant skin here and slice the meat on a mandolin for LC/keto cutlets)
- Seaweed, dried and toasted
- ACV works in this soup, to taste
- Any spices or herbs you like (Cilantro, dried basil, turmeric are all high in potassium)

Cover vegetables with water and cook on low for 2-3 hours. Replenish any water as it evaporates out.

After cooking strain out the solids and press the vegetable pulp through a strainer.

Helpful Hint: I fill quart containers, label them with the name and date and freeze them.

Pickle Juice Pops by Sandy Tucker Rodriguez:

A wonderful low carb treat on a hot summer day.

- 16 ounces of dill pickle juice, right from the pickle jar
- 2 oz. water

Mix the pickle juice with the water and place 2-4 oz. of mix into 4-6 pop molds or small paper cups. You can also use an ice cube tray and add Popsicle sticks. Freeze until hard and firm.

Helpful Hint: Add tiny hunks of chopped pickle to the mix or add a sprinkle of pink salt. No need to dilute with the water unless you find the juice to strong.

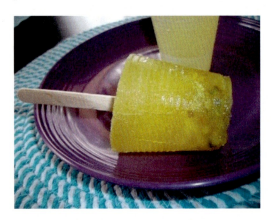

Guacamole Con Zucchini by Sandy Tucker Rodriguez:

- 1 large zucchini, diced
- 1 large avocado, diced or mashed
- ¼ cup fresh cilantro, chopped
- 1 small Roma tomato, diced
- 3 green onions, chopped or ¼ cup onion, chopped
- 1 tbsp. mayonnaise
- Salt to taste

In covered casserole dish, cook zucchini in microwave oven until tender, about 4 to 5 minutes. Drain in a strainer over a bowl to remove moisture. Meanwhile in medium bowl, mash the avocado and mix in chopped cilantro, tomato and onion. Add the cooked, drained zucchini and salt. Blend in mayonnaise. Serve with pork rinds or vegetable sticks.

Helpful hint: this recipe can be used as a topping for tacos or rolled up in ham slices for parties.

String Beans in the Greek Ladera Style by Pete Kaye:

"Ladi" is the Greek word for oil, and in Greece, olive oil is king. So, this style of cooking is called Ladera. This technique can be done with any combination of vegetables. My all-time favorite is Celery Ladera!

- ¼ cup extra virgin olive oil
- ½ onion diced
- 2-3 cloves of garlic
- 1 pound of fresh green beans trimmed and cut into bite size pieces
- 1 fresh tomato (our tradition was to peel it, but there is good fiber in the skin)
- 1 tsp. salt (I prefer Himalayan or Celtic)
- ¼ tsp. black pepper
- ¼ tsp. dried oregano

The method is the same here regardless of what vegetable you choose. Add a small amount of olive oil in the pot, add the onion and garlic until they turn fragrant.

Add the remainder of the olive oil and add the green beans. At this point, reduce the heat to simmer and cook covered for about 30 minutes.

Helpful Hint: A quarter cup of olive oil sounds like a lot, but most of the oil is absorbed into the veggies as they simmer.

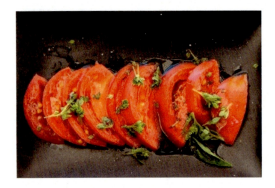

Simple Coleslaw by Sandy Tucker Rodriguez:

- 3 cups shredded cabbage(green or red)
- 2 chopped green onions
- 1/4 cup chopped green pepper
- 2 Tbsp. vinegar
- 1/2 tsp. dill
- 1/4 cup mayo
- Sprinkle Sea salt/ black pepper to taste

Mix vinegar with mayonnaise, dill, green pepper, salt and pepper. In a large bowl add chopped onions to cabbage.

Pour mayo mixture into bowl and toss over cabbage. Mix well.

Helpful Hint: This is not a sweet coleslaw. If you want it sweet use a pinch of liquid stevia

My Favorite Green Salad by Sandy Tucker Rodriguez:

- Chopped mixed greens(spinach, romaine, arugula)
- Sliced cucumbers
- Sliced red radish
- Chopped red, green bell peppers
- Whole olives
- Diced green onions
- Chopped avocados
- Chopped pecans
- Halved cherry tomatoes
- Sprinkle of feta cheese

Add what you like to your favorite salad. Toss and serve

Green Avocado Dressing by Sandy Tucker Rodriguez:

- 1 avocado mashed
- 1/4 tsp. yellow mustard
- 1/2 cup avocado mayonnaise (or any mayonnaise)
- 1 Tablespoon minced green onion

Mix well or blend in food processor. Sprinkle with sea salt and black pepper to taste.

Helpful Hint: Makes a tangy salad dressing. Refrigerate for a few hours to overnight Add more mayonnaise if you prefer a thinner consistency.

Apple Cider Vinegar Spiced Tea by Sandy Tucker Rodriguez:

- 1 cup of warm/hot water(8-10 ounces)
- 2 Tablespoons organic apple cider vinegar
- 2 slices of lemon
- 1/2 tsp. Ceylon cinnamon (optional)

Mix well and stir.

Helpful Hint: Serve warm or add ice for iced tea. I drink this in the early morning and again before bed.

Gina's 1 Week Sample Menu

By Gina More Minis

Everyone asks me about what I eat. Well, I've decided to provide a one week sample menu.

I follow a cyclical ketogenic diet, where I adhere to a strict ketogenic diet for six months, limiting carbohydrates to 20g per day. During the remaining six months, I carefully introduce more carbohydrates.

On LCHF, I don't count carbohydrates, since my carbohydrates are derived from whole vegetables. Once a week, I incorporate starches, such as tubers and squashes, or seasonal fruit. All other carbohydrates, such as grains or additional sugars, are avoided. I use salt liberally to season foods. I incorporate apple cider vinegar during each meal to aide in digestion, and drink spring water after each meal. When I begin my daily fast, it's a water fast.

Day 1

<ins>7:30 AM Breakfast:</ins>

- 2 Jones Little Pork Sausages
- 1 tbsp. butter
- 2 scrambled eggs
- 1 tbsp. salsa
- 1 tbsp. olive oil
- 1 cup coffee
- 2 tbsp. half and half

<ins>12:00 PM Lunch:</ins>

- 8 oz. sirloin steak
- 2 tbsp. butter
- 2 cups green beans
- 1 petite sweet potato
- 1 tbsp. sour cream
- 1 tbsp. extra virgin olive oil

Water fast begins.

Day 2

<u>7:30 AM Breakfast:</u>

- 1/4 cup raw pecans
- 1/4 cup raw walnuts
- 1 tbsp. flax meal
- 1/2 cup half n half
- 1 cup coffee
- 2 tbsp. half and half

<u>12:00 PM Lunch:</u>

- 2-3 cups spinach leaves
- 1 vine ripe tomato
- 4 white asparagus spears
- 2 hardboiled eggs
- 1 tbsp. apple cider vinegar
- 1 tbsp. extra virgin olive oil
- 3 boneless, skinless, thin cut, chicken breast cutlets (a little over 8 oz) coated in pork rinds and pan fried in ghee and avocado oil

Water fast begins.

Day 3

<u>7:00 AM Breakfast:</u>

- 3 bacon strips
- 2 eggs scrambled in the bacon fat
- 1 tbsp. salsa
- 1 tbsp. extra virgin olive oil
- 1 cup coffee
- 2 tbsp. half and half

<u>12:00 PM Lunch:</u>

- 2-3 cups riced cauliflower

- 2 vine ripe tomatoes
- 1 oz. feta cheese
- 2 tbsp. extra virgin olive oil
- 1/2 lb. ground beef cooked in ghee with peppers, onions, garlic and chopped tomatoes

Water fast begins.

Day 4

7:30 AM Breakfast:

- 1 vine ripe tomato
- 1 avocado
- 4 slices fresh mozzarella
- Fresh basil leaves
- 2 tbsp. extra virgin olive oil

12:30 PM Lunch:

- 1/2 lb. burger
- 3 slices cheddar cheese
- 2 cups spinach leaves
- 1 vine ripe tomato
- 1 tbsp. extra virgin olive oil

2:00 PM "Dinner":

- 1/2 bar Taza 95% stone ground chocolate

Water fast begins.

Day 5

6:30 AM Breakfast:

- 2 Jones Little Pork Sausages
- 1 tbsp. butter
- 2 scrambled eggs
- 1 tbsp. salsa

- 1 tbsp. olive oil
- 1 cup coffee
- 2 tbsp. half and half

12:00 PM Lunch:

- 1/2 lb. beef meatballs, made with cinnamon, allspice, carrot, onion, garlic, red pepper, egg and almond flour
- 2 cups riced cauliflower pilaf, made with carrot, celery, green peas and turmeric
- 1 tomato
- 2 cheddar cheese slices
- 2 tbsp. hummus
- 2 tbsp. olive oil

Water fast begins.

Day 6

7:30 AM Breakfast:

- 1/4 cup raw pecans
- 1/4 cup raw walnuts
- 1 tbsp. flax meal
- 1/2 cup half n half
- 1 small apple

9:00 AM:

- 1 cup coffee
- 2 tbsp. half and half

11:30 AM Lunch:

- 1/2 lb. beef meatballs, made with cinnamon, allspice, carrot, onion, garlic, red pepper, egg and almond flour (left over from yesterday)
- 2 cups California Blend vegetables (carrots, cauliflower, broccoli)
- 1 tbsp. butter
- 1 tomato

- 2 tbsp. hummus
- 2 tbsp. olive oil

Water Fast Begins.

Day 7 – One Meal A Day

Brunch 9:00 AM:

- 1/2 lb. ground beef, 3 eggs, onion, pepper, garlic, spinach, tomato paste baked in the oven as a frittata. I topped it with cheese and guacamole.
- 1 almond butter bread muffin from Sandy Tucker Rodriguez recipe. This equates to 2 1/2 tbsp. almond butter and 1/2 egg. I ate it with butter.
- 1 cup coffee with 2 tbsp. half and half.

Water fast begins.

Day 8 – Veggie Day

7:00 AM Breakfast:

- 3 bacon strips
- 2 eggs scrambled in the bacon fat
- 1 tbsp. salsa
- 1 tbsp. extra virgin olive oil
- 1 cup coffee
- 2 tbsp. half and half

12:00 PM Lunch:

- 3 cups roasted vegetables, carrots, cauliflower, zucchini, yellow squash, peas and broccoli
- 1/2 sweet potato, roasted
- 1 tomato
- 2 tbsp. guacamole
- 2 tbsp. butter
- 1 tbsp. extra virgin olive oil

Water fast begins.

The End

Resources:

Intensive Dietary Management:

www.intensivedietarymanagement.com

Fung Shweigh for Diabetes/Metabolic Issues inspired by Dr. Fung:

https://www.facebook.com/groups/459769974182105/

Fung Shweigh Facebook Page:

https://www.facebook.com/Fung-Shweigh-FB-Page-313446289072931/

Natural Fats and Low Carb Recipes by Fasting Fungsters:

https://www.facebook.com/groups/346760412380512/

Fasting Lowers Cholesterol:

https://intensivedietarymanagement.com/fasting-lowers-cholesterol-fasting-16/

Why Dietary Cholesterol Is Important:

https://intensivedietarymanagement.com/dietary-cholesterol-important-idm-4-2/

X Marks The Spot – Triglycerides and Coronary Disease:

https://intensivedietarymanagement.com/x-marks-spot-t2d-30/

Is Protein Fattening:

https://intensivedietarymanagement.com/protein-fattening-hormonal-obesity-xxv/

How Much Protein Is Excessive?

https://intensivedietarymanagement.com/how-much-protein-is-excessive/

Fasting and Autophagy:

https://intensivedietarymanagement.com/fasting-and-autophagy-fasting-25/

Made in the USA
Columbia, SC
16 July 2017